I0837923

The influence of changing gender roles throughout the 18th & 19th Century on the position of women in the practice of midwifery and gynaecology

By Barry Vale

Contents

Abstract

The central theme of this work will be a discussion as to whether or not changing gender roles throughout the 18th and 19th centuries influenced women wishing to have a career in midwifery and gynaecology. Midwifery in an informal sense at least has existed for thousands of years whenever women (and sometimes men) have helped other women through pregnancy and childbirth. Gynaecology as a specialist form of medicine can be traced back to the Ancient Greeks and the Romans and was traditionally dominated as a profession by men. In Western Europe gynaecology along with other medical practices had gone backwards after the fall of the western half of the Roman Empire. In the eastern half of the Roman Empire based around Byzantine such practices continued till its fall in the 15th century. The rediscovery of Greek medicine from Arabic texts translated from Byzantine books led to the re-emergence of medical treatments on a greater scale whilst linking university education with the best-qualified practitioners (Loudon, 1997 p. 61).

There will be detailed analysis and debate as to the opportunities available to women to gain entry into these two medical areas that could be of such importance to the health and well-being of women then as much as it remains so today. How such influences of changing gender roles varied from country to country will also are explored in some detail. At the start of the 18th century women, even wealthy ones had very little control over their lives and powerful women would only have such power by accident of their birth. Arguably powerlessness over their lives and opportunities would prove to spur on feminist movements to change that. Women in most societies were considered to be the fairer and therefore the weaker gender and the roles assigned to them generally reflected their perceived strengths and weaknesses. Thus many men argued that women should not learn about things that only men needed to know about or be allowed to do things that only men should do.

The reasons for depriving women of meaningful opportunities and fulfilled lives were partly social, partly economic and partly religious. At the start of the 18th century the overwhelming majority of midwives were women. The majority of gynaecologists were men even if women should be the ones most concerned about their ability to have children when they wanted them with reduced concerns about childbirth proving fatal both to them and their children. Poorer women had in reality negligible control over their own present and future (a situation that still persists in much of the Third World). While social and medical changes would arguably start to develop over the next two centuries childbirth remained dangerous both for women and their children. Economic and political changes especially in Western Europe and the United would have an impact on women and their social and employment status. There were changes in midwifery and gynaecology during this period both in terms of medical advances and the role of women within the professions, which will be fully outlined.

Introduction- background and overview

History seems to be dominated by accounts of the achievements of men in general and of powerful men in particular. In contrast the lives of virtually all women and the poorest or most common of men is either unknown or difficult to understand in great detail.

Fortunately the 18th and 19th century provided greater levels of evidence than earlier centuries, which allows for more research to be carried out (Mendelson & Crawford, 1998, p.1).

If observing the world in 1700 the lack of power women had to control their own destinies seems starkly apparent (even in some parts of the world that is the case in the present day). Men, the men who wielded power and influence were often drawn from the social and economic elite and did not wish to share it with men of lower status and women of any status, dominated the world in all aspects. That is not to say that women were not considered useful or important, rather that they should be confined to the traditional gender roles that they were given to perform or so thought the ruling male elite (Mendelson & Crawford, 1998, p.1).

Women depending on where they lived had few or no legal rights, restricted or non existent career and educational opportunities having often to rely on male relatives as well having to be supported by male relatives. Poor women often had to work in the poorest conditions in jobs that required no or the merest level of education and offered no prospects. In that respect they were probably in a similar position to working class men especially unskilled labourers although of course even the lowest paid men were determined to be paid more than women (Eatwell and Wright, 2003, p. 207).

In 1700 only a few women could achieve positions of power and even gain education or careers yet they were the exception rather than the rule. Some countries proved more enlightened to others when it came to extending the roles and responsibilities that women were allowed to perform (Eatwell and Wright, 2003, p. 207). Husbands could even deprive their wives of a midwife during labour as they had the legal right to do so (Mendelson and Crawford, 1997 p. 4).

There were certainly profound social, economic and political changes that changed many aspects of women's lives most notably from the late 18th century. These changes and developments that were in essence continuations of some earlier trends that can be traced back to the 15th and 16th centuries if not earlier. These changes also had an effect upon men, which did not always favour the women that were attempting to improve themselves and further their opportunities. Men were often concerned with their own prospects rather than those of women (Hobsbawm, 1962, p. 1).

Aside of being born into nobility, the upper classes or royalty women found it difficult to have control of their own lives let alone anyone else's. Even women in these privileged positions were often held back from independent action by traditional cultural and social norms of behaviour. Women rulers such as Catherine the Great of Russia could show ruthless ability yet was considered exceptional and masculine in quality. Catherine the Great was probably the most effective ruler that Imperial Russia had after Peter the Great. She did not however make any attempts to change Russian society and change any of its gender roles, leaving the vast majority of Russian men and women illiterate and ignorant. In Britain although only a constitutional monarch, Queen Victoria was regarded as being a paragon of virtue, a woman that always carried out her duties without fuss and maintained all the traditional gender roles that a wife and mother were supposed to carry out (Gardiner & Wenborn, 1995, p.818).

Queen Victoria and those around her tended to portray the royal family as a fine example of a traditional family with traditional values not only in Britain but across its vast Empire as well. The British monarchy was all in favour of conserving society just as it was to maintain its prestigious status although it was the elected government that carried out policies intended to conserve or to transform society. The British Royal family could also set trends as with the use of obstetricians and man midwives such as William Hunter to deliver their children. Countries such as France gave women no property rights at all whilst in Britain women only had property rights before they got married. As by and large English law had be transported across with the original English colonists the United States had very similar laws relating to women rights in Britain (Gardiner & Wenborn, 1995, p.818).

Given the lack of midwifery and gynaecology available and the poor knowledge of the medical issues surrounding pregnancy and childbirth it should come and no surprise that the mortality rates of women and children were so high. Once knowledge about gynaecology and midwifery improved it contributed to the lowering of infant mortality rates. For poor women the only kind of medical service they would receive was those that were provided by family and friends or less enthusiastically by the workhouses. Midwives then as now only help with straightforward births. Gynaecologists when they could be afforded would increase but not completely ensure the survival of mother and child. Any complications could often result in the death of mother and child (Youngson, 2000, p.489).

From the 18th century there began a decline in the infant mortality rates in Western Europe and North America that would eventually lead to changes that would alter the lives of women there. Women often had larger families to allow for the fact that many children died in infancy and because they did not have contraceptives available to them. Having children as long some of them survived to adulthood was also the best means of being looked after when people grew too old to work and wished to avoid the workhouse and the shame of a pauper's grave (Gardiner & Wenborn, 1995, p.414).

Whilst some population growth as a healthy sign of a nation's wealth and possibly its military strength others believed that increasing populations only made nations poorer. Poverty so Thomas Malthus contended in his 'Essays on Population' kept the population growth under control as well as keeping the poor in their rightful social and economic positions. Going against the conventional wisdom of the era Malthus contended that having larger families made people poorer (Hobsbawm, 1962, p.238).

Ironically enough middle class and wealthier families did start to have fewer children as the cost of caring for and educating them increased alongside the decline in infant mortality that meant more children lived on to become adults. Reducing the size of families meant that women would not have to spend so many years looking after their children thus increasing their availability to go out and work. Of course women from wealthier families had more options in that children could be looked after by nannies or sent to boarding schools (Hobsbawm, 1962, p.238).

 When considering the opportunities of women becoming midwives it has to be remembered that not all women held official positions. Carrying out unlicensed midwifery could get women into trouble although Parish Councils and magistrates often tolerated these women as they worked amongst the poorest and their wages frequently kept them from falling into the workhouses themselves. Midwives work was not always just confined to assisting the delivery of children sometimes it included looking after orphans (Mendelson and Crawford, 1998 pp. 284-85).

Chapter 1

The influences of the French Revolution and the Enlightenment

The 18th century and especially the 19th century would witness changes that would affect the status of women that were eventually reflected in the practice of midwifery and gynaecology. The prevailing social attitude at the start of this era was that women were inferior to men, an attitude that may have remained intact at the end of the era yet did not go unchallenged by women and a few male supporters of increasing women's rights and opportunities. Even the upsurge of liberal thought that resulted from the French Revolution only regarded liberty, fraternity and equality for men. Radical thinkers such as Jean Jacques Rousseau still considered women as being less physically and mentally able as men (Schama, 2002, p.74).

There is much to suggest that French women lost ground to men as a result of the French Revolution. This was mainly due to middle class and to a lesser degree working class men gaining a greater say if not actual control in running the country solely to serve their own purposes as women were barred from the political process (Mendelson & Crawford, 1998, p.1).

Men experiencing political participation for the first were not about to give women a taste of influence if not actual power immediately. Besides if they thought about such issues at all they would have believed that if middle and working class men improved their economic and social position then that would also improve the lives of their wives and children. Considering France was at the forefront of giving men rights and equality in many respects it lagged behind other countries in giving women better opportunities and changing legal inequalities. The majority of French men seemed content with their social, economic and legal gains that followed from the French Revolution that they felt no real need to change things (Roberts, 1997, p.95).

However some medical developments did occur as a result of the

French Revolution that would eventually contribute to changing gender roles and allowing women to have opportunities for careers in gynaecology and midwifery. Under the monarchy of the Ancien Regime public hospitals had been controlled mainly by the Roman Catholic Church or privately run by medical guilds. In 1794 the French government took control of all hospitals with all doctors, surgeons and midwives being controlled by the state if not always directly paid by it (Loudon, 1997 p. 319).

State control of medical services was primarily intended to improve France's ability to wage war by keeping people healthier and to ensure that there were enough boys to become future soldiers or sailors and industrial workers. It was also essential to ensure that there were enough healthy girls to maintain population growth by having healthy children themselves. That was not a change of gender roles just the placing of greater emphasis on existing ones. In other words a healthy nation would have the ability to be a great military and economic power whilst an unhealthy nation would become weaker. The French revolutionary and imperial governments were just as concerned with the threat posed by Britain, Russia and Prussia as its royal predecessors were along with the possibility of being encircled by them (Roberts, 1997 p. 121).

The French Revolution led to changes in the French education system that in theory should have helped France become a major economic and military power as well as changing gender roles. As a result of the French Revolution the French government established the Ecole Nationale and the Ecole Polytechnique to produce world class economists, engineers and surgeons. Places at these elite schools were almost exclusively preserved for the most capable male students around. Women found it very difficult to gain entry to them. The schools did help the French to become experts in medical and engineering fields, even more specialist than prior to the French Revolution. It was a paradox that the French Revolution preached the gospel of equality yet produced an education system that continued to produce elite specialists rather than educate all girls and boys to a universally high level. The education system tended to reinforce elitism rather than introduce equality or lead to the changing of gender roles. Conversely though the two- tier system of healthcare in France did allow the opportunity for women to become medical practitioners. In economic terms it meant that French concentrated on quality rather than quantity and could not match the growth of Britain, Germany and the United States which may also explain why gender roles changed at different rates in these countries (Hobsbawm, 1962, p.177).

Women tended to receive less education than men did although illiteracy rates amongst the poorest were almost universal. Women from wealthier backgrounds tended to have their education greatly restricted in comparison to their male counterparts. Generally they were only taught enough to be good wives and mothers. It was little wonder then that there were so few women involved in midwifery and gynaecology or other professions that required any education at all (Gardiner & Wenborn, 1995, p.818).

 For many women the harshness and often the brevity of life excluded them from attempting to gain separate identities or careers for themselves. Not only did women give up property that they owned upon marriage, high death rates during or after childbirth meant that women were more likely to die young than their husbands (although men had fairly low life expectancy as well compared to modern averages in Western Europe and North America). It was not uncommon for men to remarry two or three times and outlive all of their wives (Roberts, 1996, p.208).

There are indications that women were more likely to live longer if they had fewer children. As there was little effective forms of contraceptives and no abortions during this period the best ways to control the number of children was to settle down later on in life or to remain celibate which was rarely a viable option. Some European countries such as France had governments that wanted the population of their countries to keep increasing. Europe at this time was starting to experience strong population growth that went closely in hand with economic development and was inter linked with social and cultural changes (Roberts, 1996, p.208).

Women had been disadvantaged in their gender roles since ancient times because men regarded them as being less physically and mentally capable. Studies of gynaecology and anatomy convinced men that women's bodies were strange and unusual, even Aristotle had found women a mystery. Men have traditionally being reluctant to allow women to have control of their own bodies. It was not just Jews and Christians that saw women as potential temptresses bringing about the downfall of unwary men (displaying moral double standards that infuriated many women). Gynaecology maybe all about the female body yet it was a field of medicine that men were determined to retain control of throughout the centuries. Women were blamed for leading men astray, spreading sexually transmitted diseases and were often left literally holding the baby if things went wrong for them (Porter, 2001, pp.104-05).

The more complicated gynaecological procedures were not routinely performed until the end of the 18th century. Gynaecologists like the majority of doctors in other areas of medicine generally wished to avoid the most difficult procedures unless they were the best qualified. Gynaecologists had to consider that there was not guarantee that their patients would get infected or die through shock or blood loss. Major surgery of any kind was only usually attempted if not operating would kill the patient anyway. New medical practices were often developed by travelling surgeons that charged higher fees and would operate when other doctors dared not. The 19th century began with gynaecology featuring the greater use of operations such as hysterectomies. Medical advances meant that more women were treated yet it meant that medical treatment became more expensive. Improvements in gynaecology were certainly made more bearable for women undergoing treatment through the use of pain relieving anaesthetics. Such advances also meant that women became more interested in pursuing gynaecology as a career (Porter, 2001. pp.218-19).

Chapter 2

The impact of social and economic changes

Women had started to witness their gender roles and lives being affected by social, economic and religious changes during the 16th and 17th centuries. Some changes tended to help women whilst others seemed to hamper their progress towards making their lives better and inadvertently changing gender roles. The emergence or more accurately the growth of the middle class in countries such as Britain, France and Germany would cause and accelerate changes in gender roles particularly in the 19th century. Out of the political tumult that followed in the wake of the French Revolution would emerge the first feminist movements (Eatwell & Wright, 2003, p.207).

Mary Wollstonecroft would provide much of the arguments and impetus for such movements through 'A Vindication of the Rights of Women' first published in 1792. Wollstonecroft argued that women were equal to men in worth and ability yet were deprived of that equality through the actions of a male dominated world. Women were much more that just wives and mothers (Schama, 2002, p.74). A Vindication of the Rights of Women was a sound foundation for the movements that would eventually improve the opportunities that women had to receiving education and aim towards meaningful careers. Mary Wollstonecroft did not survive the birth of her second child who went on to become the famous author Mary Shelly (Gardiner & Wenborn, 1995, p.817).

Mary Wollstonecroft was part of an increasing number of women that had refused to be wives, mothers or daughters and nothing else. These women were similar to the trade union or working class movements amongst men that aimed at self- education as a means of improving their lives.
Women had other things in common with the working class men, low pay (if they had a job) and being denied the vote. Whilst there were campaigns in some countries to give all men the votes the calls to give women the vote aside from John Stuart Mill were few and far

between (Morgan, 1993, p.515).

In countries like Britain women's interests were not represented and hardly ever discussed. Moves towards political reform were generally aimed at getting all men the vote (Hobsbawm, 1975, p.102). The 19th century did however witness legal reforms in Britain that when combined with social and economic changes improved the status, rights and opportunities that women held. Women were given rights to keep their property after marriage, divorce was made easier to obtain and women were given rights of custody over their children. Reforms such as these allowed more women to gain control of their destinies and contributed to a gradual change in gender roles. Women slowly gaining entry into the education and medical professions amply demonstrated that such changes were taking place (Gardiner & Wenborn, 1995, p.818).

The level of education available to women and men varied from country to country throughout the 18 and 19th centuries. In all countries the great majority of the well educated were men. There were disparities in the rate of illiteracy across the world. The great bulk of the peasantry in countries such as Russia, China and India remained illiterate en masse. In contrast countries such as Sweden had virtually an entire population that was literate. Where women were better educated became the places where changed in gender roles were strongest. The growth of literacy that strengthened throughout the 19th century was promoted for various reasons. The Industrial Revolution meant that men and women who worked in factories needed to be literate and numerate to be effective workers that could stay safe. The expansion of secondary and university education in the United States and Germany helped them to further their industrial and economic development (Hobsbawm, 1975, pp.42-43). However, it was the expansion of primary education that was most noticeable in Western Europe in the last decades of the 19th century in France, Britain and Germany. Across Europe as a whole the population increased by a third yet the number attending school increased by 145 per cent (Hobsbawm, 1975, p.95).

While midwifery and gynaecology had been professions around for centuries another profession that was to be dominated was to emerge inadvertently. That profession was nursing during the Crimean War of 1854-56. The British contribution to that war was notable for its military ineffectiveness and the collapse of even it usual primitive military medical treatment. Florence Nightingale became the heroine of the war and nursing became suitable for middle class women to have greater employment opportunities (Roberts, 1996, p.357). Mary Seacole in fact provided the most successful nursing and medical treatment. Her popularity with the troops was not reflected in the media, unlike Florence Nightingale she was black and not from a middle class background (Schama, 2002, p.220). There were a large number of women that became nurses during the bloody American Civil War of 1862-65 although their numbers were soon reduced after the war finished. Women also proved their worth as nurses during the Franco-Prussian War of 1870-71 (Hobsbawm, 1975, p.142).

Chapter 3

The emergence of Obstetrics and Man midwifery

The growth in popularity of maternity or lying in hospitals led
reflected the general increase in hospital construction and led to an
outpouring of books and teaching on midwifery and childbirth. Such
books and teachings showed the greater knowledge of the childbirth
process acquired and shared by William Smellie, John and William
Hunter plus other contemporaries.
The teachings and writings of William Smellie amongst others
helped to make midwifery, gynaecology and obstetrics attractive and
popular professions. Smellie himself had originally studied in Paris.
His work would ensure that these subjects would be studied in
London and his home city of Edinburgh not to mention a host of
other European universities and hospitals. The brothers John and
William Hunter also came from the Edinburgh area and would prove
just as influential on the development of gynaecology and obstetrics.
John Hunter had studied the development of embryos, which
increased the understanding of how babies developed before birth
and the best ways to deliver them safely (Loudon, 1997 p. 210).

John Turner was a key innovator in the study of surgery and medical
experiments based on dissection allowed for a greater understanding
of the human body. He studied a wide range of areas including
midwifery, anatomy and pathology. John Turner's work certainly
raised the level of knowledge available to gynaecologists,
obstetricians and midwives not to mention dentists and those treating
sexually transmitted diseases (Porter, 2001 p. 225).

William Hunter was an accomplished surgeon teaching surgery and
anatomy in London hospitals or in the academy he ran with his
brother John. William Hunter refined the practices and procedures
of obstetrics; it was largely his efforts that got it recognised as a
distinctive branch of medicine. From being a man midwife he went
along way in his career. Such was his renown that he delivered the
children of George III and Queen Charlotte thus increasing the
profile and popularity of gynaecology, obstetrics and man midwifery
amongst the middle and classes. This no doubt in turn increased the

numbers wanting to pursue a career in gynaecology or midwifery (Crystal, 1998 p. 472).

The lying in hospitals allowed more students to carry out obstetrics procedures and provided better care for women especially poorer ones. The hospitals did not at first prove much safer than home deliveries especially as women did and their children were more likely to die of infections. The 18th century saw the opening of many new hospitals across Europe and the United States. London for instance increased its capacity to treat hundreds of patients to 20,000 patients at any time. London overtook Paris as the best centre of medical studies with Edinburgh also gaining a reputation for excellence. London trained more men midwives than anywhere else did, or accouchers as they liked to describe themselves. Some doctors took the accouchers training courses to add to their medical skills and combine delivering babies with their other roles as general practitioners (Porter, 2001 pp. 214-15).

These accouchers not only had a sound knowledge of anatomy, they were linked to maternity hospitals and they were able to use forceps during difficult childbirth. Wherever possible gynaecologists, obstetricians tried to avoid caesarean sections as they increased the dangers for women. Men midwives and gynaecologists could also consult new books on the subject. Perhaps the most outstanding book of this type was William Smellie's 'Treatise on the Practice of Midwifery' of 1752. Not only was the text of the highest quality the accompanying pictures were extraordinarily detailed and realistic, almost photographic in quality. The increasingly level of knowledge and skills were certainly a great benefit to women as more of them survived and fewer of them lost their children. Smellie did not just confine his work to theory, for instance he developed new more effective forceps that offered less risk both to mother and child. Smellie would not charge poor women for their medical treatment if his students were allowed to attend the births and gain hands on experience (Porter, 2001 p. 225).

Smellie advised that all midwives should have a complete understanding of anatomy prior to taking up their positions. He did not mind if midwives were men or women as long as they were mature and dependable. The book also gave advice on changing the traditional rituals of washing children after birth to reduce the amount of broken bones and bruising. He also recommended a thorough examination of children to check for any injuries or illnesses. The effectiveness of midwifery could be increased and its costs reduced by keeping every procedure simple and straightforward (Smellie, 1752 Volume I, Book 4 Chapter II).

 In the countries with better levels of midwifery and gynaecology available infant mortality reduced markedly by the end of the 19th century and in the early part of the 20th century. If the Netherlands is compared to backward Russia the difference is obvious. In the 1870s, 200 out 1000 Dutch children did not reach their first birthday compared to 260 Russian children, by 1914 the respective figures were 100 and 250 (Hobsbawm, 1987 p. 193).

Chapter 4

Religious and Secular influences

Before the onset of the period under discussion in this dissertation there had been educational and scientific developments that laid the foundations of changes in gender roles that would eventually allow some women opportunities in midwifery and gynaecology. The Renaissance had stimulated the growth of education and the search for knowledge (Mendelson & Crawford, 1998, p.1).

The impact of the Renaissance and the Reformation was to be increased by the use of printing and the adoption of vernacular languages that would eventually allow common men and women greater opportunities. An unintended outcome of this was to be the 16th century Reformation and Counter Reformation that affected the gender roles of women in Western Europe and the areas of North and South America that these Europeans gained control of in this period (Loudon, 1997 p. 195).

The Reformation had prompted further growth in the provision of education although it did not have such beneficial effects on the availability of health services. Even teaching ordinary people to read the bible in their own language had considerable consequences which if underestimated now were certainly recognised at the time. Whilst in Protestant countries women no longer had the opportunity to join Convents they did have more chances to have a basic education in order to read the bible and be able to read it to their children. Although Protestants often had a conservative view of society and the role of women within that society they inadvertently furthered capitalist and educational development. Protestantism affected education and society differently in different countries, contributing for instance in the provision between Scotland and England. Scotland giving women slightly better chances of gaining a decent standard of education (Chadwick, 1990, p. 173).

The Reformation had caused the closing down of hospitals as well as schools attached to or run by monasteries or convents. Sometimes those hospitals were reopened whilst others remained closed. Aside from London new hospitals had not started to emerge in most parts of Britain until the 18th century. The wealthier members of society could afford to pay for private medical, midwifery and gynaecological services although the standard of services could vary in quality. For the poor the availability of such services was not always guaranteed. The Elizabethan Poor Law Act of 1598 and 1601 still provided the framework for paying for doctors, nurses and midwives for the poor (Chadwick, 1990, p. 173).

Parish Councils usually decided on which doctors and midwives to use, their decisions often based on saving ratepayers money as much as professional qualifications and abilities. However, the system usually operated smoothly without much incident or scandal. Such a system gave women opportunities in nursing and midwifery even if it did not change roles enough to let them become gynaecologists. Medical treatments were normally carried out at the patients' home although that changed to hospitals and workhouses with the Poor Law Amendment Act of 1834 (Loudon, 1997, p.195).

Women in Protestant countries found it difficult to change gender roles within their societies especially where more fundamentalist or Puritanical Protestantism was strongest. To justify their unfair and sometimes harsh treatment of women the Puritans used biblical quotations and their interpretations of scripture. As far as the fundamentalist Protestants were concerned the Bible was not only literally true and of greater factual merit than science or the study of nature and people. The real clincher was that the Bible was divinely inspired and any roles assigned to men and women by it should not be altered in any way at all (Chadwick, 1990, p. 174).

Women in general and Eve in particular had been responsible for mankind falling from grave and the expulsion from the Garden of Eden. For the Puritans Eve's part in the Original Sin was the raison d'être for making women subordinate in all social, economic, legal and religious matters. The Bible also implied that women held a subordinate position to men as man had been created first. The Puritans saw good and bad things as a sign of God's favour or anger, ideally the Godly prospered and sinners were punished. Arguably women suffered pain during childbirth as a consequence of Eve's actions; God punished all women for the sin of the first one (Mendelson and Crawford, 1998 pp 32-33).

Some Puritans in England were unhappy with the Church of England for not been forceful in maintaining the subordination of women, as it should have been. The English Puritans unhappy with the Church of England eventually separated from the national church or immigrated to the American colonies although more serious political and religious differences than the gender roles of women caused that rupture. That immigration contributed to the Puritanical nature of some parts of United States society (Mendelson and Crawford, 1998 pp 32-33).

Not all the Protestant sects were convinced of the inferiority of women or that gender roles were set in stone because that was how they should be because that was the way it had been done in the Bible. The Society of Friends more commonly referred too as the Quakers believed that God had forgiven humanity for the Original Sin. As a result of that divine forgiveness women were no longer being punished by God and therefore should be punished by men. Thus the Quakers allowed women greater control and autonomy over their own lives as they were not mentally or morally inferior to men even if they not as physically strong as men. The Quakers and the greater responsibilities and roles they encouraged women to perform undoubtedly contributed to the changing of gender roles (Mendelson and Crawford, 1998 pp 32-33).

Women especially poorer or working class women tended to marry later than those from wealthier families did. Women from such backgrounds were more likely to work before they got married as their families were more likely to need their pay to get by on. They were more often employed as domestic servants were, or in cottage industries and later on in expanding industries or public services such as teaching or midwifery. Poorer couples tended to delay marriage so that they could save money so that they could afford to have their own separate home and not have to live with one family or the other (Mendelson and Crawford, 1998 pp 32-33).

Building up savings was also done for when the wife had to give up work to look after their children or if the husband found himself unemployed or under-employed. Women preferred to get married as it gave them a higher social status than remaining single. However the difficulty in obtaining divorces and the lack of employment opportunities to married women meant that 'they were more likely to feel impelled to make marriage work as a social and economic partnership' (Mendelson & Crawford, 1998, p.131).

Although women were taught to obey their husbands, not all women chose to do so without question. Women with a more forceful character could have a greater influence upon their husbands and were more likely to have daughters that questioned the permanence of gender roles (Mendelson & Crawford, 1998, p.135).

Chapter 5

The growth of education and the emergence of role models

Demands for the provision of education for women grew throughout this period especially in the 19th century. Some wished for better - educated women just make them better wives and mothers (Mendelson & Crawford, 1998, p.1).

Women were showing signs of wishing to have a better education that made them useful members of society rather than just good cooks. Women were already able to have careers in midwifery and gynaecology in France, where unlike Britain they were not barred from obtaining degrees. It was in the maternity wards of Paris that Emily Blackwell became the United States second women doctor (Schama, 2002, p.244).

The first women doctor in the United States was actually her sister Elizabeth Blackwell. The Blackwell sisters opened women's dispensary in New York in 1856 and were involved in the London School of Medicine for Women (Crystal, 1998, p.112). The first woman in Britain to qualify as a doctor was Elizabeth Garret Anderson who graduated in 1865 despite there being a great deal of opposition to women becoming qualified doctors rather than just nurses. Elizabeth Garret Anderson was determined to allow other women to pursue medical careers without the struggle that she had faced to get a university place. Therefore she helped start to change gender roles by opening a dispensary that offered college courses in London. That dispensary was later turned into a hospital for women named after Elizabeth Garret Anderson following her death (Crystal, 1998, p.29).

Elizabeth Garret Anderson was only able to open her dispensary and hospital through the funding given by her husband who made a fortune as a ship owner. Men were not entirely willing to allow women to change their gender roles so women mostly had to do that for themselves. The establishment of medical colleges for women to study medicine, nursing, midwifery and gynaecology was a great step forward. It was an advance as they could get the training they

needed to become doctors, nurses, midwives and gynaecologists.
The provision of university and college education for women prior to
this was sparse at best and could depend on which country women
aspiring towards higher education lived in or could afford to move to
study in (Schama, 2002, pp. 246-47).

Through much of the 18th and 19th centuries university education
remained expensive and was largely for the sons of the wealthy.
Even when women had been able to attend lectures and found the
time and money to study at university or college they were not
always been allowed to sit exams and therefore their studies with no
formal qualifications. The advent of women's colleges resolved the
problem of women not been able to study and sit exams yet did not
immediately reduce male prejudices against women trying to gain
access to professions that men had always controlled and dominated.
Women such as Elizabeth Garrett Anderson and the Blackwell
sisters plus the women that followed in their footsteps drew ideas for
their personal and professional development from a source that may
not at first seem obvious. That source of inspiration was Charles
Darwin and his book the 'Descent of Man' that was first published in
1871. It caused as much debate yet not as much controversy as the
infamous 'Origins of the Species had done. Women could and did
use the Descent of Man to inspire the ascent of women. Following
Darwin's theory women aiming to achieve something meaningful in
their lives believed that the key to progress lay in sound education
and hard work (Schama, 2002, pp. 246-47).

Both the Enlightenment and advances in natural and social sciences
pointed towards the progression of the human race, yet much of that
progress only appeared to favour men plus a few privileged women.
For ambitious women education would allow them to become better
people and more suitable for work that benefited their societies.
Women were not naturally inferior to men and they had it in their
power to gain equality with men and be the fittest of the species.
The women that followed in the footsteps of Mary Wollstonecroft
realised facts that men had known for a long time, the effective use
of knowledge and only restricted access to that knowledge had
meant that men could get all the best jobs and be paid the most.
Knowledge equals power whilst the gaining of knowledge can hold

the key to individual empowerment. For women having no control over the provision of midwifery and gynaecology services was tantamount too not been in control of their own destinies (Crystal, 2003, p. 252).

Women were left out of the Enlightenment movement that was only intended to achieve progress for men and not women. It was Enlightenment movement that furthered secularisation of society thus altering social and economic relationship within Western Europe and the United States. The leading figures of the movement such as Voltaire, Hume and Jean Jacques Rousseau were not noted for their approval of increasing opportunities for women in midwifery and gynaecology or in any other areas. However with much of its influence upon some government policies and Western Europe plus its contribution to the French Revolution it played its part in changing gender roles (Abercrombie, Hill & Turner, 2000, p.119).

Chapter 6

The Impact of Industrial Changes

Women started to gain greater education opportunities towards the middle and the end of the 19th century, which in turn helped increase their employment opportunities. Changes in the economies of industrialising countries meant that poorer women had lost jobs in traditional cottage industries such as cotton spinning to find work in factories and later in the new schools, offices or hospitals .

The Industrial Revolution had been funded by more effective agricultural production especially in Britain and to a lesser extent in France. The greater availability of food reduced infant mortality and contributed to the increasing rate of population growth in Britain and other parts of Western Europe. An increase in population meant that there was a greater need for gynaecology and midwifery services although that was of course dependent on how poor women were. The 19th century saw a steady growth of government involvement within the provision of education, social and health services. Such increases provided women with further opportunities to gain meaningful careers and further change gender roles (Morgan, 1993, p. 477).

Hand in hand with industrialisation in Western Europe at least went urbanisation that also had an impact on the changing of gender roles that helped women forge careers in gynaecology and midwifery during the 18th and 19th centuries. The expansion of the cities increased the need for even the most basic of medical treatments. The high demand for poor relief and medical treatment strained the poorhouses of France and the workhouses of England almost to breaking point. Whilst the cholera epidemics that spread across much of the globe from the 1840s prompted the greatest building of sanitation infrastructure since the end of the Roman Empire (Gardiner and Wenborn, 1995, p. 156).

Perhaps it was no coincidence that women got their best chances to become qualified doctors, nurses, midwives and gynaecologists in major cities such as London, Paris and New York. Britain in this period witnessed the great expansion of towns such as Birmingham, Manchester and Glasgow into major cities in their own right. For these cities were in greater need for trained medical staff than most other places. Nursing and midwifery were usually seen as more natural professions for women to enter as they were caring professions and women were generally considered to be more caring than men are.   On the other hand gynaecology like other branches of medicine was widely considered by male medical practitioners to be beyond the capabilities of women to understand. Women were increasingly allowed to work in hospitals, medical practices or surgeries due as much to the lack of qualified men as much as a realisation that they were in fact capable of doing anything men could do (Porter, 2001 p.312).

Women were seen as cheaper substitutes for men. Even when their presence was needed it was not always welcome. Medicine was as prone to gender discrimination as much as any other area of employment. Women were paid less across the board than men were for social and economic reasons that developed faster under a capitalist system. Women were only expected to work until they got married from which point their husbands were supposed to support them whilst they stayed at home and raised any children they had and carried out all domestic chores. Gender roles did not change, as quickly as many women would have hoped. To put things in perspective only a tenth of married British women worked in 1911 (Hobsbawm, 1987 pp 198-99).

The French Revolution led to a revolution in French medicine as well and French politics and society. The old royal French system had been complicated in structure, very elitist in nature and virtually impossible for women to become involved in practising any type of medicine. Under Napoleon there was a two- tier system of health care provision. There was the fully licensed that included all the medics that had passed their degrees. The lower order had either not completed all their exams or had failed them and were only allowed to practice on the poor. It was this second lower tier of medical practice that would allow women to become gynaecologists and other types of doctors. These medics learnt their trade by treating the poor that lived in the poorhouses or used them as a last resort. The doctors of these poorhouses were backed by nursing assistants that had m included as part of their duties. The use of nursing assistants to do m duties was not really a reflection of changing gender roles (Porter, 2001, pp.312-13).

The only things that had changed was that they now worked for the French government rather than the Roman Catholic Church and that rising urban population meant that none of them were needed. The biggest change in gender roles came as women were allowed access to the second tier of medical practitioners that allowed them to take gynaecology or obstetrics. By hard work women were given the glimmer of opportunity to become fully qualified doctors even if it did take years of working in poorhouses. French medical practices were transported to Germany as a result of the Napoleonic Wars. This system allowed for the treatment of the poor yet was not very caring for them at all (Porter, 2001, pp.312-13).

The French had started to regulate their doctors, gynaecologists, nurses and midwives before the French Revolution and tightened up control afterwards. The Germans were equally keen on such regulation of medical professionals. Britain and the United States were slower to regulate their gynaecologists and midwives. State regulation was not a bad thing for women in that it could allow them to become gynaecologists and midwives providing that they could meet the minimum criteria (Porter, 2001, pp.312-13).

All these countries an expansion of their hospital services that generally offered women greater opportunity to become gynaecologists and midwives to cater for rising populations and expectations of higher levels of medical services. At the turn of the 20th century the United States seemed to be swimming against the tide when the gender roles were changed to the detriment of women. Women midwives were removed in favour of men that formally at least, better qualified. However that move to men midwives proved unsuccessful. Women midwives were brought back (Porter, 2001 p. 325).

In other parts of Western Europe the midwife traditions and profession was much better developed than in Britain in general and in England particularly. The Germans, the Scandinavians and especially France took a much greater interest in midwifery. That is not to say that British women involved were any less capable than their continental contemporaries just that the British government took less notice of the issues surrounding midwifery (Loudon, 1997, pp.207-09).

Women in Britain as in most other countries had nearly always performed midwifery, although during the 18th century there was a change in gender roles that disfavoured women rather than help them. The 18th century witnessed growth in the availability of medical services and an increasing trend towards using men midwives rather than women. This was partly a fashionable trend and a way of social showing off, as men cost more than women did.

As the 19th century went on the trend was to go back to women midwives in Britain. It was found out that men midwives were no more effective than women midwives and there was always an element of moral ambiguity in allowing men to be close to women during and after childbirth (Loudon, 1997, pp.207-09).

The 18th century was to witness fairly profound changes in a branch of medicine closely linked to gynaecology and midwifery, that of obstetrics. Obstetrics would eventually help lower infant mortality and reduce the number of women that died as a result of childbirth. Obstetrics and midwifery services increased in availability with noticeable acceleration during the last decades of the 18th century. The presence of doctors present at births to midwives advice or take over deliveries should there be an emergency went from an insignificant number to between 30-50 per cent of births by the end of the 18th century. Knowledge of pregnancy and childbirth had hardly improved since antiquity until the 18th century. Medical text-books from the 17th century or earlier would not be much use to modern day gynaecology and midwifery students yet those of the 18th century are just about at the modern level of knowledge and would not require much adaptation to be useful. Perhaps one of the finest books from the 18th century was an 'essay on Natural Labour'. This seminal study of the stages of labour was written by Thomas Denman and was first published in 1786. As knowledge of obstetrics grew more men wished to become involved in delivering babies than before as gynaecology, obstetrics and man midwives (Loudon, 1997, p.209).

Life in the 18th century could still be a struggle for women especially poor women yet there were grounds for optimism, the lives of women would get better and that such improvements would eventually allow them greater chances to succeed in having a better influence and position within their society. The expansion of capitalism especially in Britain generated more wealth that went towards funding education and health services. The new wealth was not of course evenly distributed with the already rich and the newly rich gaining the most and not always sharing it. Increased wealth can help to explain previously mentioned in gynaecology and midwifery care provided (Black, 1997, pp.153-54).

 More money meant that more gynaecology and midwifery could be paid in theory allowing evidence of women taking part more frequently in public life that can be argued demonstrates that there was changing gender roles. It is not always easy to judge how much of those changes were actually new areas of change or already existent changes reported or noted for the first time. Of course the rate of changes in wealth and gender roles was not uniform, some cities or regions saw faster, deeper changes than others did. For instance London witnessed more changes than Edinburgh did whilst Edinburgh witnessed more changes than most rural areas of Britain. Social trends could demonstrate that women could effectively handle any extra opposition and responsibility that changing gender roles could offer them. Women certainly become more visible during the 18th century, be it in theatres performing plays or in the fashionable coffee -houses and tea -rooms which the London Debating Societies seemed to prefer. However it would be misleading to argue that women were on the brink of equality with men or about to achieve economic and social parity. It was one thing for men to talk to women in tea-rooms it was not likely that they would willingly women a greater influence upon their own opportunities (Black, 1997, pp.153-54).

Chapter 7

National and Ideological influences

In the majority of cases any changes in gender roles that leaped women gain within the gynaecology and midwifery favoured women from wealthier backgrounds through the 18th and 19th century and beyond. Women societies and economies then as now offer the greatest opportunity to the rich who are already in a better position to exploit their chances. The 18th century had witnessed the continued rise in literacy levels that had started in the 16th century yet only women from wealthy backgrounds or those from middle class backgrounds improved their levels of education on a par with men (Coward, 1997, p.87).

Protestantism was full of paradoxes that assisted transitions in social and economic fields as well as political ones that were not always intended to happen. Protestant emphasis on hard work and sobriety were seen as a means for men and to a lesser extent for women to improve their lives by being able to support themselves and avoid debt or the workhouses. Education was seen as a vital means to r salvation as well as a means of improving job prospects. Protestants were more likely to educate their daughters to make them more useful family members. Education was only supposed to keep men and women in their respective gender roles yet making them perform all tasks more effectively. Such e activity played its part in promoting capitalism, which proved a catalyst for major social and economic changes. Capitalism can be regarded as the key element of gradually making the societies of Western Europe and North America more secular and materialistic in outlook (Coward, 1997, p.87).

Secular societies were more likely to generate changing gender roles albeit with continued resistance from men that did not wish to yield too much ground to women. Secularism and materialism did not automatically mean that men deliberately changed gender roles for the benefit of women to allow entry into professions (Schama, 2002, pp. 246-47).

Instead secularism and materialism helped to nurture the ideologies of socialism and communism. Neither socialism nor communism was intended to improve the position of women. Their sole purpose was to improve the position of the poor and working class men which would coincidentally improve the lives of women they were related to yet that was only a by product of equality between men. Socialism and communism did however help women to work towards changing gender roles. Some women saw their inequality as being solvable by using socialist or communist approaches whilst other women believed that they had to change things for themselves. For these latter women liberal, conservative, social and communism were just different methods men could use to control the lives of women (Eatwell and Wright, 2003 p. 208).

Although many women saw Communism (although it was usually referred to as Marxism) as a male dominated ideology like al others it did have the benefits of allowing feminists to analyse the gender differentiation within societies. Marx had not paid attention to the position of women within societies though Engels tried to rectify that fault during the 1880's (Abercrombie, Hill & turner, 2000, p.118). Communism did not however contribute to any major changes within gender roles during the 18th and 19th centuries. Contributions to changing gender roles came during the 20th century with the Communist regimes of the Soviet Union and China. Whatever the other merits or failures of the Soviet Union it certainly produced more women doctors, teachers or engineers than had previously existed (Abercrombie, Hill & Turner, 2000, p.328).

For women becoming gynaecologists was harder than becoming a midwife as a university degree was needed. Midwifery was a profession that was more accessible for women than gynaecology especially in Britain and United States were was no formal regulation of standards, qualifications and recruitment until the 20th century (Abercrombie, Hill & Turner, 2000, p.328).

Changing gender roles so those women could attend university and gain degrees was probably the most important change that allowed women entry to a career in gynaecology. However, as previously mentioned access to university for men let alone was restricted to the wealthy unless the potential student could gain sponsorship or a scholarship. Similarly access to primary and secondary education had been restricted in most parts of Western Europe until the middle of the 19th century. Throughout all schools within this period boys and girls were rigorously separated from each other in different schools (Abercrombie, Hill & Turner, 2000, p.328).

Boys usually being taught subjects that would help work in industry or commerce, whilst girls were normally taught things that would help them carry out more feminine careers and be useful at a domestic level. Just how important education was and is in shaping or changing gender roles or other social norms can be ascertained by the struggles between the Church of England, Non-Conformist Protestants and the Roman Catholic Church to fund schools and control elements of the curriculum. Similar disputes occurred in France and Italy over whether the Roman Catholic Church or the state should decide and control what children learnt at school. Tight controls of subject matter at schools may have been meant to prevent the spread of radicalism yet it also aimed at conserving existing social structures (Coward, 1997, p.87).

In England throughout the majority of this period university education was denied to any potential student who was not a member of the Church of England following the Restoration of the monarchy in the 1660s. The Non-Conformists had got around that ban by establishing Dissenting Academies that did not ban women from studying at them. The removal of restrictions on university places to non-Anglicans may have had a limited effect on changing gender roles yet men were undoubtedly the main beneficiaries of such moves (Coward, 1997, p.87).

 As there were considerably fewer university graduates during the 18th and 19th centuries as there are not gaining a degree had a great deal more prestige then. A degree could make all the difference between an average career and a highly successful career. Whilst women were only slowly gaining access to university some found that if they had a good basic education that they were more likely to marry a graduate with a better job and more money. As the differential between men's pay and women's pay remained great it made more practical and economic sense for women to find well paid husbands rather than trying to build their own careers and having their own independent income to use as they saw fit. During this period men justified their higher wages with the argument that they had to support their wives and children. There was widespread social stigma attached to families in which the wives had to go work as it implied that their husbands were failures. However the stigma of a wife having to work was almost certainly better than going to the workhouses for assistance and the almost inevitable breaking up of the families forced to do so. The emergence of housewives was a feature of 19th century societies and was related to the end of cottage industries that had allowed women to earn extra income yet stay at home (Hobsbawm, 1987, p.198).

Women not only found it difficult to find work with equal pay they often found that they had to settle for jobs of lower status. Women were less likely to join trade unions than men were and those that did found that the trade unions were more focused on the issues those men regarded as being important. The only trade unions where women formed the majority of members were teaching, nursing and midwife ones. Even when trade unions had a large number of women members' men almost without exception dominated its leadership. Employers and trade union leaderships dominated by men were frequently willing to make the working conditions of women worse than those they would tolerate for themselves were (Black, 1997 p.235).

Conclusions

Therefore overall changing gender roles did affect the ability of women to pursue careers in gynaecology and midwifery during the 18th and 19th centuries. The affects of changing gender roles were not however uniform across the globe or indeed throughout this two century period. In most societies women held inferior social, economic, legal and religious positions than men did at the start of the 18th century which was reflected in their inability to gain the means to further their careers and ambitions. In the vast majority of cases such inferiority of position remained there at the end of the 19th century and continued into the 20th century.

Up to the 18th century the knowledge and practice of gynaecology and midwifery had not advanced at all in centuries, women were already performing as midwives although gynaecology effectively remained closed to them, as they could not go to university. Gender roles did not change overnight; they were the result of a combination of various factors. Changes in religious and secular beliefs and practices had an impact on social and economic developments that in turn contributed to further changes in gender roles. At the start of the 18th century much of Western Europe and North America were still Christian in belief and religion was seen as more important than is the case today. Christianity had a strong influence upon culture and the forming of gender roles. Protestant and Roman Catholic Churches alike regarded women having an inferior position to that of men although with various ideas about how rigidly defined gender roles should be.

Protestants were more prone to being fundamentalists and believing that gender roles should as much as possible be based on Biblical pronouncements on the matter. Protestantism in some ways contained elements that made it contribute to changing social and economic situations even if its intentions were to preserve the good and transform the bad things within the societies that held influence over. Protestantism emphasised that it was up to the individual to improve his or her life that hard work would be rewarded by a better standard of living and laziness would bring the workhouse nearer. When enough people did work hard or invest wisely it brought capitalist developments that altered the opportunities available for women although not always for the better.

Greater wealth was not shared out evenly yet gender roles did start to change as women from middle class backgrounds believed that they could wok as well as fulfilling their roles as mothers, wives or daughters. The profile and effectiveness of gynaecology, obstetrics and midwifery had been enhanced by the achievements of William Smellie along with John and William Hunter. For students of midwifery William Smellie's books and course if they could afford to buy them were a revelation in the best theory and practice available.

Whilst women such as Elizabeth Garret Anderson and the Blackwell sisters tried to and eventually succeeded in gaining entry into the medical profession the position of women in midwifery had been threatened with the growing fashion for the man midwife. That fashion was mainly confined to Britain yet it did reduce the opportunity for women in midwifery. Man midwives were even officially introduced into the United States to replace all women midwives at the start of the 20th century.

 In Britain women would regain the majority of midwife positions and went on to take advantage of employment opportunities in other areas such as nursing, teaching and office work. Overall women did gain from changing gender roles yet those changes only slowly filtered through into better opportunities in gynaecology and midwifery or any other professional occupation for that matter. Gender roles changed with varying degrees from country to country although women were still a long way from achieving equality or succeed in having many of them become gynaecologists in 1900 at the end of the period studied.

Bibliography

Abercrombie N, Hill S & Turner B S (2000) Penguin Dictionary of
Sociology 4th edition, Penguin, London
Black J (1997) A History of the British Isles, Macmillan Press LTD
Basingstoke
Chadwick O (1990) The Penguin History of the Church 3 – The
Reformation, Penguin, London
Coward B (1997) Social Change and Continuity: England 1550 –
1750, Longman, London and New York
Crystal, D (1998) The Cambridge Biographical Encyclopedia,
Cambridge University Press, Cambridge
Crystal, D (2003) The Penguin Concise Encyclopedia, Penguin,
London
Eatwell, R. & Wright, A (2003) Contemporary Political Ideologies
2nd Edition, Continuum, London
Gardiner J & Wenborn N (1995) The History Today Companion to
British History, Collins & Brown, London
Hobsbawm E (1962) the Age of Revolution 1789-1848, Weidenfeld
and Nicholson, London
Hobsbawm E (1975) the Age of Capital 1848-1875, Weidenfeld and
Nicholson, London
Hobsbawm E (1987) the Age of Empire 1875-1914, Weidenfeld and
Nicholson, London
Loudon I (1997) Western Medicine – An Illustrated History, Oxford
University Press, Oxford
Mendelson S and Crawford P (1998) Women in Early Modern
England, Oxford University Press, Oxford
Morgan K O (1993) The Oxford Popular History of Britain, Oxford
University Press, Oxford
Porter R (2001) Cambridge Illustrated History Medicine, Cambridge
University Press, Cambridge
Roberts, J.M (1996) A History of Europe, Penguin, London
Roberts J M (1997) The French Revolution, Oxford University
Press, Oxford
Schama S (2002) A History of Britain 3 – The Fate of Empire 1776-
2000, BBC Worldwide, London
Smellie W (1752) A Treatise on the Theory and Practice of

Midwifery, 3 Volumes, D Wilson, London
Youngson R (2000) The Royal Society of Medicine Health
Encyclopedia, Bloomsbury, London

Midwifery, 3 Volumes, D Wilson, London
Youngson R (2000) The Royal Society of Medicine Health
Encyclopedia, Bloomsbury, London

www.ingramcontent.com/pod-product-compliance
Lightning Source LLC
Chambersburg PA
CBHW051134250726
48655CB00007B/3052